bullied, not broken

WHEN THE BULLIES DON'T WIN

nate neustadt

Limit of Liability/Disclaimer of Warranty: While the publisher and the author have used their best efforts in preparing this book, they make no representations or warranties with respect to the accuracy or completeness of the contents of this book and specifically disclaim any implied warranties of merchantability or fitness for a particular purpose. No warranty may be created or extended by sales representatives or written sales materials. The advice and strategies contained herein may not be suitable for your situation. You should consult with a professional where appropriate.

Published by: LiveFullOut Media, LLC

www.bulliednotbroken.com

A portion of the profits of every book is donated to the Born This Way Foundation, which supports the mental and emotional wellness of young people.

ISBN: 978-0-578-55258-3

Library of Congress Control Number: 2019911050

dedication

I dedicate this book to Whoever you are. Wherever you are. I kept you in my mind the whole time. I don't know if you're in elementary school, high school or even college, but I wrote this for you.

If you've been picked on, targeted by other kids for whatever reason, I wrote this for you to give you hope. To help you realize that you're not alone and to arm you with the tools and mindset to fight back. That doesn't mean physically attacking those who are picking on you or treating them in the same awful way they're treating you. I want to give you something far more important than that: the knowledge that you're not alone and that there's help out there and how to get it. And that you will be stronger for this experience. I promise.

Whether you're a boy, girl, straight, gay, transgender or bisexual. Whether you love theatre, or sports, or math. Whether you're outgoing or quiet and thoughtful. Whether you're tall, short, thin, overweight, with clear skin or have zits. Whoever you are. Wherever you are. Because bullies can target anyone, and anyone can become a victim.

This book is for you.

contents

"Bullies are scared people hiding inside scary people."

– MICHELLE OBAMA

introduction

One in four kids are bullied in the U.S.[1] In fifth and sixth grade, I was the one. I was a victim of cyber, physical, and verbal bullying. I was called hateful names and made fun of because of my appearance and the things I love outside of school. I was kicked, pushed and got awful text messages and videos.

It made me anxious, gave me a constant stomach ache, affected my participation in class and my grades, and made me not want to go to school. So I know what it feels like, and how much more awful it can make it if you don't tell anyone and you feel like you're alone. I'm here to tell you you're not alone.

I wrote this book because I want to share my story with you, and the story of others a lot older than I am who have had huge success. Because I want you to know that you'll get through it, and that there's a whole lot to learn from the awful pain.

That's not the only reason I wrote this book. I'm Jewish, and as I'm typing, I'm 13 and preparing for my bar mitzvah. If you don't know what that is, a bar or bat (for girls) mitzvah is a religious ceremony in Judaism. When Jewish boys turn 13 (or girls at 12 or 13), they go through a process of studying the Torah and learning how to lead a religious service. It also marks the age when, according to Judaism, we become a man or woman under Jewish law and tradition and are responsible for our actions and decisions.

Part of the process of becoming a bar or bat mitzvah is doing a service project. It took me a long time to figure out what I wanted to do. Really long. I'm talking two years long. After a lot of thinking, I decided I had to do something that was really personal to me. I wanted the benefits of my project to go on long after my bar mitzvah. I also love to write (journalism has been my absolute favorite class), and I know from my parents' success as authors that books impact people long after they're written.

So I decided I had to write a book about bullying, and I wanted the profits to go toward a non-profit focused on increasing awareness and providing resources to kids going through it. I've chosen Lady Gaga's Born This Way Foundation, because I admire and am inspired by her messages to be ourselves and stand up and stand out for what we believe in. Her foundation is doing powerful work, and I'm proud to support it. There are a lot of people doing great work on this issue and trying to help. I've included a list of Helpful Resources at the end. But it takes all of us standing up, speaking up and helping each other to stop bullying in all of its forms.

You're likely reading this because either you want to better understand bullying or you've experienced it or maybe you're an adult who works with kids or has kids going through some tough times. I hope one day I'll get to hear your story, but until then, you should know mine.

In fifth grade I started at a private school to get away from Common Core Math and classes I'd be a bit more interested in. The school I started going to was supposedly the best. I had to take tests and interview to get in, so my parents and I were excited when I got accepted. It was a *big* deal. When I got there, the first couple weeks were good, and I thought I was making some cool new friends.

But I learned more about people at that school than anything they taught me in my classes. I learned that just because someone's smart, doesn't mean they're nice. By the middle of September, I started getting teased. At first it was because the kids in the class said a fellow classmate and I were boyfriend and girlfriend, even though we weren't.

They'd constantly tease us at school and on a class text loop. I was so embarrassed. I mean it was hard enough being the new kid in a small class that had been together for years, let alone having the spotlight shone on me with a girl that I barely knew.

But it didn't end there. Our math teacher would have us grade each other's papers. It was hard for me to adjust to Singapore math, and most of my homework wasn't right.

My classmates would tease me for getting so many answers wrong. After class one day, one of the kids said to me, "You're not smart enough to be here."

That really hurt and confused me because I went through the same admissions process as everyone else. It was like Warner telling Elle in *Legally Blonde* that she wasn't smart enough to be at Harvard Law when she had to take the same LSAT and do the same application process. So I stopped raising my hand because I didn't want to appear stupid, which I now can see looking back was the really stupid part. I wasn't getting the help I needed to understand our math lessons. My grade took a nosedive, along with my self-confidence.

When my math teacher reached out to my parents to talk about my poor grades, my parents sat me down for a talk. That's when I finally told them I was being teased, and that's why I was so quiet and sucking at math.

My teacher talked to the whole class about the importance of asking questions, which gave me a safer space to learn. It was clear that had I gone to my teacher and my parents earlier, I could've avoided so much stress, the nosedive my grades and feelings took, and weeks of feeling like a loser. Things got better...until January.

After winter break, I returned to school and a new set of challenges. I was getting kicked and punched by a group of girls in my class. One of them was actually the girl who I'd been "coupled" with in the earlier teasing.

They'd pick on me I'd be in the hallway, at recess and even in the classroom (they'd figure out ways to tease me without the teacher seeing). During lunch I'd hide in a part of the campus I knew would be safe. I'd sit by myself, just waiting for lunch and school day to end. I hated going to school and the stress was giving me stomach aches every day.

I tried to deal with it on my own. I did what most kids probably do. I talked to the kids. I told them to stop. I tried to act cool and tried to fit in. I acted like it didn't hurt. But no matter what I did, it continued. I didn't hit back because I've always believed boys and men shouldn't hit girls or women.

I didn't say anything to my parents, teachers or school administrators because I didn't want the kids to get in trouble. Yep, I was more concerned about them than I was about myself, and I thought if I told on them, they for sure wouldn't ever like me. And I didn't want to make waves in this school that everyone said I was so lucky to get into. I didn't want to upset my parents because they said this was the best school and how amazing it was that I got in.

I learned that I wasn't the only one getting bullied. One of my friends was getting beaten up in the bathroom by boys in the other fifth grade class. He was so full of anxiety his mom would have to come pick him up early from school.

This went on until March, until I couldn't take it anymore.

I came home from school one day, threw my backpack across the room and yelled, "I can't stand it!" My parents asked me what happened and that's when I told them. I pulled up my pant leg and showed the huge bruise on my shin. "Remember the girl who the other kids thought was my girlfriend? She was wearing boots and kicked me in the shin as I walked by her desk." I told them everything that had been going on since January.

And that's when the you-know-what hit the fan. To make a long story short, my parents got way involved, and when the head of school and the dean of students didn't take this all as seriously as my parents thought they should, they pulled me out of that school and into a new one. For the second time in less than a year, I was once again the new kid.

Normally my new school didn't let kids come in midyear. But my dad called the head of admissions and explained the situation, who then called an emergency entrance committee meeting. Two days later I started at my second new school, which I love. Two years later, I'm still there and am now the class student council representative.

I immediately felt included and made friends the very first day. I felt safe to ask questions, make mistakes, and be totally me. I finished fifth grade without stomach aches and anxiety, with a new set of friends and so much excitement about starting middle school.

But here's what's interesting. Anyone can have a great class full of friends and still get bullied at school. When I was in sixth grade, it was a group of seventh graders who decided I deserved to get picked on. And I started not wanting to go to the school I loved.

I'm the shortest in my class by a lot (thank you very much, short ancestors), and these boys were calling me "dwarf" and "midget" and making fun of the size of my feet. And because I'm into musical theatre and acting and take dance classes to one day be "a triple threat" and increase my chances of success in show biz, they called me "fag", "faggot" and "gaylord".

I was super scared. I thought for sure what happened to me at my other school was happening all over again. Except this time I thought it would be worse. I'd never before been called "faggot" and I knew it was a hate word.

Again, I asked them to stop. They didn't. I asked them again. They didn't. I even yelled and cussed at them because I got so angry.

Luckily, I didn't keep quiet this time. I told my parents, and I told the dean of students. The school was diligent and dealt with the problem very quickly. The bullying stopped for a while, but then the boys started teasing me again. This time they also called me "tattle tale." I'd learned before that keeping quiet doesn't help, and even if the kids started being mean again, it just meant that I had to ask for help again.

I talked to my parents and again went to the dean of students. Turns out I did the right thing. Because I spoke up, it led to a larger investigation, which uncovered that these kids were teasing a lot more people. It wasn't just me getting bullied. The school took it very seriously and made sure it stopped. I don't know exactly what they said to the students, but none of us have been bullied again. It was great to know that speaking up helped not just me, but other kids too. Lesson learned.

Things can change, and it can get better. But it requires the one being bullied to speak up as soon as it starts happening. I think that I would've spoken up a lot sooner if I didn't on some level think there was something wrong with me. There must be something wrong with me for other kids to do and say such awful things. That's a whack way of thinking, but I bet you've thought it, too.

But here's the reality. First, if someone is bullying you, they're likely bullying others, too, and if you keep quiet, all of you will suffer. We found out that the girl who had been kicking and punching me in fifth grade had picked on other kids too. And the seventh-grade boys were spreading their verbal harassment far and wide.

Second, the bullies are the ones who have something wrong. And they're likely hurting more than you. The punching/kicking girl's parents were getting a divorce, and her whole life was changing. Now just because she was hurting she didn't have the right to hurt anyone else, but it shows it wasn't about me or her other victims. And I have to imagine those seventh graders on some level didn't feel super confident about themselves if they felt they had to tear down others to feel good.

And third, while I wish the bullies had dealt with their feelings better, I learned that I can't control them. I can only control myself. These experiences made me more committed to the things I love that I was teased about because I refused to back down from being me. It's made me more empathetic for others who are bullied, discriminated against and suffering, and made me passionate about helping them.

Well, that's my story—what I've been through and what I've learned. Now I'm excited to share with you 19 more.

I researched successful and famous people who were bullied, and I'm excited for you to read what they've been through and how it made them stronger and influenced their lives. I know there are countless stories of bullying out there, and it hurts just as much whether you grow up to be famous or not. But I picked the following people because I respect them and what they've accomplished, and they've been open about their experiences.

And a note, I refer to them by their first names not because we're buds and hang out all the time, but because I thought it would be easier to read and remind all of us that they're just people like you and me. Except for President Clinton. He's always President Clinton because he was a frickin' president.

I hope my story, and their stories, inspire you to stand up for yourself. To not let anyone stop you from doing what you love and being true to who you are. To know that you are not to blame. It's never your fault when someone picks on you. There's no excuse for bullying or bullies. It's always their fault. There is something wrong when someone has to make other people feel bad so they can feel good. And I hope they get help.

But mostly, I hope you learn from this book that you're not alone. That there is help and hope. That you can get past this and go on to do amazing things in your life.

Don't become like the bullies. Rise above them. Each one of us can still make the world a better place. We can create the happiness we want to see in the world. Talk to each other. Accept each other. Be excited for all of our differences, because the world needs a lot of different ideas and talents. The world needs your talents and your passions. Never forget that.

#1

justin timberlake

Singer, Songwriter, Actor, Author, Entrepreneur

Justin Timberlake was born January 31, 1981 in Memphis, Tennessee. He started singing and acting at a young age. When he was 11 years old, he competed on the television show *Star Search*. He didn't win, but he didn't give up on his dreams. The next year he became a cast member of the *Mickey Mouse Clubhouse*.

His epic career continued to grow. He was in the mega-hit group NSYNC, a group that sold more than 70 million records. After NSYNC he launched his solo music and acting career. He's one of the world's best-selling musicians of all time. During his solo career he's sold more than 32 million albums and 56 million singles and has received ten Grammy Awards, four Emmy Awards, seven American Music Awards, nine *Billboard* Music Awards, and eleven MTV Video Music Awards. All this and he's not even 40 yet (which is when my mom tells me things really start to get good). And this section wouldn't be complete if I didn't mention his crazy good comedic chops he's shown during his hilarious skits with BFF Jimmy Fallon and his many appearances on *Saturday Night Live*.

It's easy to look at someone like him who seems to have it all—good looks, mad talent in many areas, a talented and successful wife—and think that he always had it all and that life has always been super easy.

But I've learned that you don't get to be Justin Timberlake without a lot of hard work and experiences that make you stronger and work even harder. When Justin was a kid he wasn't celebrated for his talent and passion. He was picked on because of it and called all sorts of names. In 2010, as a guest on *The Ellen DeGeneres Show*, he talked about being called names. "If you didn't play football, you were a sissy...I got slurs all the time because I was in music and art.

"Everything you get picked on, or you feel makes you weird, is what essentially is what's going to make you sexy as an adult," he said. "Growing up in school, no one ever called me anything close to an innovator, they called me different, they called me weird, they called me a couple of other words I can't say on TV."[2]

In 2017, when he received an iHeart Radio Award, he dedicated it to kids who might be bullied or shunned. "If you are black or you are brown or you are gay or you are lesbian or you are trans — or maybe you're just a sissy singing boy from

Tennessee," Justin said to a crowd that was going nuts. "Anyone that is treating you unkindly, it's only because they are afraid, or they have been taught to be afraid of how important you are. Because being different means you make the difference. So f— 'em."[3]

What I learned from Justin:

Even if you aren't the coolest kid or you don't fit in, don't be afraid to be you. Because being different will help me make a difference.

What did you learn?

_____

_____

_____

_____

_____

"You always have to remember that bullies want to bring you down because you have something that they admire."

- ZAC EFRON

#2

tyra banks

Model, Game Show Host, Actress, Entrepreneur

Tyra Lynne Banks was born on December 4th, 1973, in Inglewood, California. Tyra began her career as a model at the age of 15. She was the first African American featured on the covers of *GQ* and twice on the *Sports Illustrated* Swimsuit Issue. She was a Victoria's Secret Angel from 1997 to 2005. In the early 2000s, Tyra was one of the world's top-earning models.

She began acting on television in 1993 on *The Fresh Prince of Bel-Air* and has had small roles in movies and TV series including *Gossip Girl* and *Glee*.

In 2003, Tyra created and began presenting the long-running reality television series *America's Next Top Model*. Tyra also had her own talk show, *The Tyra Banks Show*, which aired on The CW for five seasons and won two Daytime Emmy awards for Outstanding Talk Show Informative. In 2017 she became the host of *America's Got Talent*, where my family enjoyed watching her.

In 2010, she published a young adult novel titled *Modelland* based on her life as a model. It became a *New York Times* Best Seller. Tyra is one of only four African Americans and seven women to have repeatedly ranked among the world's most influential people by *Time* magazine.

Tyra's experience with bullying started with her being the bully. At around ten, she would fight a lot with her brother, which he almost always won. She ended up taking her frustration out on girls at her small private school, being the "mean girl" and excluding girls from the clique she led and insulting them.

The tables turned on her when Tyra moved to a large public school. It's hard to believe one of the most famous and successful supermodels and TV personalities of all time was bullied because of her appearance, but it's true. "When I was 11 years old, I grew three inches and lost 30 pounds in three months. So I went from being a mean bully, cute little chubby girl to shooting up, weighing 98 pounds and just looking sick and frail," Tyra said.[4]

"I wasn't sick, but people thought there was something wrong with me. I was the brunt of every joke, every bad thing. I hated my reflection in the mirror. I would try to stuff food down my throat to gain weight," she said, adding that people called her "lightbulb head" and "five head" because she had a big forehead as a kid.

The bad memories still live with her. "Even though I later gained weight and became a supermodel, that girl always lived inside of me and I know what that felt like," Tyra said. "Experiencing the pain of being picked on turned me around. It turns out that the best things [to happen to me] in my life were to have no friends, and to be made fun of every single day," Tyra said in a *Teen People* interview.[5]

"The girl that is ripping you into shreds, is the girl that is hurting more than you ever could," Tyra said in an interview with *Popstar!*. "She's insecure, she has issues and she's ripping you to shreds because she's crying inside. I know it hurts when they say these types of things, but just know that she got some problems."

What I learned from Tyra:

Bullies are sometimes lashing out because they've been hurt too. So it's more proof that it's not about you, the one being attacked. There's something going on in the life of the bully that's making them do these awful things.

What did you learn?

_____

_____

_____

_____

_____

"Bullying happens because weak people need to prop up their ego by beating up or humiliating others."

- BRUCE DICKINSON

#3

steven spielberg

Director, Producer, Entrepreneur, Philanthropist

Steven Spielberg was born December 18, 1946 in Cincinnati, Ohio. He's one of the most successful movie directors, producers and entrepreneurs ever. He directed blockbusters like *Jaws*, *Indiana Jones*, *E.T. the Extra-Terrestrial*, *Jurassic Park*, *The Color Purple*, *Schindler's List*, *The Post*, and *Ready Player One*.

Steven co-founded DreamWorks Studios (now Amblin Partners) and was the producer for movies such as *Back to the Future*, *Men in Black* and *Transformers*. He's won three Academy Awards. His films have grossed more than $10.1 billion worldwide.[6]

But when he was younger, Steven was verbally and physically bullied. His family had moved to Phoenix, Arizona and they were the only Jewish family in their neighborhood. He was targeted because of his religion, because he was a self-described nerd and because he played in the band and orchestra.

He faced a lot of anti-Semitism. Steven was called "a dirty Jew" and was beaten up after school. Kids sneezed "a-a-Jew", mimicking a sneezing sound, as he walked past them. In a *New York Times* article, he said, "In high school, I got smacked and kicked around. Two bloody noses. It was horrible."[8]

As a result of the constant bullying, the man behind such classics as *Jaws*, *E.T.* and *Schindler's List* said that for a long time he "denied" his Judaism. "I often told people my last name was German, not Jewish," Steven shared. "I'm sure my grandparents are rolling over in their graves right now, hearing me say that.

"It wasn't so much that I wanted to be popular or wanted to meet girls," he told a *New York Times Magazine* reporter. "I just didn't want to get hit in the mouth."[9] Fortunately, when he was a teenager, he discovered filmmaking, which changed his life and touched the lives of millions and millions of people who have enjoyed and been inspired by his movies. "I had found a way to accept myself in my own life by making movies," he said. "I found that I could do something well."[10]

Steven's philanthropic efforts are jaw-dropping, and it's easy to see a connection to the attacks he felt growing up. After he made *Schindler's List*, Steven started several foundations to support the Jewish community and survivors of the Holocaust (which was bullying on the most horrific, catastrophic scale).

The Righteous Persons Foundation was created from

the profits of *Schindler's List* to grant money to Holocaust memorial efforts. He began the Shoah Foundation (Shoah means Holocaust in Hebrew) in 1994 to document Holocaust survivors and "capture the real stories from not only the individuals who lived it (mainly the Jewish population), but also those who experienced it first-hand such as gypsies, homosexuals and other minorities that were affected by the Nazi regime."[11]

In researching Steven and his life's work, I was most taken with what *The New York Times Magazine* reporter, Stephen Dubner, took away from their time together. He wrote that in a serious conversation with Steven, "'tolerance" and "intolerance" are among the most common words to crop up. Despite his success, he says, he still feels like an outsider, forever stamped by his childhood. His movies add up to one long argument for tolerance, a plea to accept the outsider.

What I learned from Steven:

The hurt I experience as a kid can be the fuel I use in my life to make a real difference, even on a huge scale.

What did you learn?

_____

_____

_____

_____

_____

#4

william (bill) clinton

**42nd President of the United States,
Governor of Arkansas, Philanthropist**

William ("Bill") Jefferson Clinton was born William Jefferson Blythe III on August 19, 1946 in Hope, Arkansas. He served as Governor of Arkansas twice, from 1979-1981 and 1983-1992. When he first became Governor, he was 32 years old, the youngest Governor in the nation at that time, and the youngest ever in Arkansas. In fact, he looked so young, he was often called the "Boy Governor."

He was elected the 42nd President of the United States and served two terms. During his presidency (1993-2001) our country had the longest period of peacetime economic expansion in American history. President Clinton left office with the highest approval rating of any president since World War II.

After he left office, President Clinton created the William J. Clinton Foundation, which works on issues including the prevention of HIV/AIDS and global warming. In 2009, he was named the United Nations Special Envoy to Haiti. After the devastating earthquake in Haiti in 2010, President Clinton teamed up with George W. Bush to form the Clinton Bush Haiti Fund. He's been married since 1975 to Hillary Clinton, a former Senator from New York, former Secretary of State during the Obama administration, and democratic nominee for President in 2016.

Anyone looking at President Clinton's modest and hard beginnings, would never have believed that he'd end up as the President of the United States. In middle school, President Clinton was picked on over and over again for being a "fat band boy" with a bad taste in clothes.

At a school dance, an older student teased him about his carpenter's jeans and punched him in the jaw! But President Clinton didn't give the bully what he wanted. As he shares in his autobiography, *My Life*, President Clinton recalls that he didn't fight back or back down, refusing to give the bully what he wanted. "I had learned that I could take a hit and that there's more than one way to stand against aggression."

He survived the bullies, and his status as a "band geek" paid off. President Clinton became a talented saxophone player in addition to his life in public service.

What I learned from President Clinton:

I learned that his bullying set him up for great success as President and set him up for the brutality of politics.

What did you learn?

_____

_____

_____

_____

_____

"When people point out your weaknesses, that's just another opportunity for you to rise above."

- ZAC EFRON

#5

jessica alba

Actress, Author, Entrepreneur, Model, Political Activist

Jessica Marie Alba was born April 28, 1981 in Pomona, California. Her father was in the Air Force, so her family moved around a lot, finally settling back in California.

She began acting in television at 13 years old and has appeared in more than 40 movies and television shows. Her first recurring television role was on the Nickelodeon comedy series *The Secret World of Alex Mack*. At 19, she became the lead actress in the television series *Dark Angel*, for which she and received a Golden Globe nomination.

She's appeared in the movies *Fantastic Four* and *Fantastic Four: Rise of the Silver Surfer* and *Good Luck Chuck*. She won the Choice Actress Teen Choice Award and Saturn Award for Best Actress on Television.

In 2012 she jumped into the world of entrepreneurship, co-founding The Honest Company with Christopher Gavigan.

The company focuses on eco-friendly and natural baby products and home goods. The company launched a line of household goods, diapers and body care products, and did $12 million in sales in its first year.[12] Jessica made Forbes 2016 list of "America's Richest Entrepreneurs Under 40," coming in at number 34.

Jessica also works to create political change. She's spent time in Washington, D.C. lobbying Congress to pass the Safe Chemicals Act. She's advocated for gay rights and worked with nonprofits including Habitat for Humanity and the National Center for Missing and Exploited Children. She's also the author of the New York Times Best Seller, *The Honest Life*.

Jessica has devoted a lot of her adult life to fighting for awareness of the causes she cares about. But when she was young, she had a terrible time fitting in at school.

Her family didn't have as much money as others in her class. She had a Texan accent and buck teeth. She was considered uncool and was frequently attacked for being different. Jessica was so afraid at school that she'd spend lunches in the nurses' office. It's where she felt safe. Her dad had to walk her to school so that she wouldn't be picked on by bullies.

Jessica never fought back, deciding that she didn't want to lower herself to the level of her bullies. But she was frustrated and scared, and she needed an outlet for those feelings. That's when she started taking acting classes.

"The idea that for an hour I could be someone different was amazing," Jessica said. "I was determined that this was something I was going to be good at. This was a part of my life no bully could ruin." She says that her lessons at drama school "changed everything" and sparked a life-long love of acting.

Jessica encourages others who have been bullied to use fear as fuel: "You have to make it push you to become a stronger person, in whatever way that may be."

What I learned from Jessica:

Don't let the bullies get in the way of doing what you love.

What did you learn?

_____

_____

_____

_____

_____

"Remember this: They hate you because you represent something they feel they don't have. It really isn't about you...So smile today because there is something you are doing right that has a lot of people thinking about you."

- SHANNON L. ALDER

#6

michael phelps

Competitive Swimmer, Philanthropist

Michael Fred Phelps II was born June 30, 1985 in Baltimore, Maryland. He's the most successful swimmer to ever live. As a competitive swimmer, Michael earned 28 medals. He's won the most gold medals ever (23). He won eight of his gold medals in a single Olympics in Beijing, China in 2008.

When you count other major international competitions, such as the World Championships and the Pan Pacific Championships, he's won more than 80 medals.

In addition to his medals, he's been named the World Swimmer of the Year eight times and American Swimmer of the Year 11 times. Because of his incredible performance at the 2008 Olympic games, Michael was named Sportsman of the Year by *Sports Illustrated* magazine. He also holds world records, including the fastest times in the men's 100-meter butterfly, 200-meter butterfly, and 400-meter individual medley.

I first saw Michael swim and win medals in the 2008 Olympics. But when I was watching him receive his gold medals, smiling on top of the podium and the US National Anthem playing, I never would have imagined that he'd been bullied as a kid.

Michael looked different and sounded different from other kids. He had long arms, a lisp and his ears stuck out. In an NBC Sports show profiling him, they reported that he had it tough at school and had talked about being taunted over his "sticky-out ears," lisp and long arms. He felt deeply hurt.[14]

Michael also struggled with Attention Deficit Hyperactivity Disorder (ADHD) and was put on medication for two years as a child. His kindergarten teacher even once told his mother, "He's not gifted. Your son will never be able to focus on anything." Boy, did he prove him wrong.

Michael was featured in the documentary *Angst*, which is about people's struggles with anxiety and depression. "If something was bothering me that would start to come out, and I would start feeling angry or depressed or upset, I would almost ignore it," he said. "I would shove [the feelings] even farther down so I wouldn't have to deal with it, so I never had to talk about it."

But he realized what I learned, and I hope you do too. That keeping the thoughts and feelings inside doesn't help. It just makes things harder. "I finally got to a point where, it was my tipping point...I started talking about the things I went through and once I opened up about that and things that I had kept inside of me for so many years, I then found that life was a lot easier," Michael said.

For Michael, the pool was a place to release all his energy and unleash his frustrations. If kids picked on him on dry land, he'd make sure nobody could stay with him in the water.

"I kind of laugh at it now," Michael said. "I think it made me stronger going through that."[15]

What I learned from Michael:

Even if you look, sound and learn differently you can still become the greatest you can be.

What did you learn?

_____

_____

_____

_____

_____

> **"Bullies are always to be found where there are cowards."**
>
> – MAHATMA GANDHI

#7

christian bale

Actor, Philanthropist

Christian Charles Philip Bale was born on January 30th, 1974 in Haverfordwest, Wales. He made his movie debut at just 13, when he was cast in the starring role of Steven Spielberg's *Empire of the Sun*. He has an incredibly long list of film credits and has earned a number of nominations and awards, including an Academy Award for Best Supporting Actor. I first got to know him as Batman, which he played in *Batman Begins*, *The Dark Knight*, and *The Dark Knight Rises*. I was even more blown away by his acting in *The Big Short*, and I'm looking forward to being old enough to watch *American Hustle* and *The Fighter*, for which he won his Academy Award. Christian is also an activist and supporter of environmental causes including the Sea Shepherd Conservation Society, Greenpeace and the World Wildlife Fund.

The boy who grew up to be 6'2" and viewed as one of the greatest actors was bullied as a kid.

In an interview with the *Mirror* in 2008 he said the attacks started after his breakout role in the *Empire of the Sun*. "I took a beating from several boys for years. They put me through hell, punching and kicking me all the time."[16]

Christian felt what I have felt and what so many bullying victims feel too. "You begin to wonder what you can change about yourself and your life to make them stop. You don't know who to talk to and what to do about it.

"Who the hell knows why it happened. People might say the bullies are jealous, but I can't explain it."

He attributes those years of misery with giving him the determination to succeed in the acting world. In fact, he said his decision to fight for a role against Leonardo DiCaprio was informed by the strength he gained during those years of bullying.

"I was not going to be bullied out of the part, I was going to stand up for myself and fight," Christian said. The part he got was in the hit *American Psycho*, which made him a huge star.

"So when I look back, problems in childhood can make you into the man you become."

What I learned from Christian:

I will get to use the strength I had to build during the time I was bullied to fight for the things I want in my life.

What did you learn?

_____

_____

_____

_____

_____

> "If they don't like you for being yourself, be yourself even more."

– TAYLOR SWIFT

#8

taylor swift

Singer, Songwriter

Taylor Alison Swift was born on December 13, 1989, in Reading, Pennsylvania. Taylor started writing songs when she was 12 and moved to Nashville, Tennessee at the age of 14 to pursue a career in country music. She signed with the label Big Machine Records and became the youngest artist ever signed by the Sony/ATV Music publishing group.

Her 2006 debut album peaked at number five on the *Billboard* 200 and spent the most weeks on the chart in the 2000s. The album's third single, "Our Song," made her the youngest person to single-handedly write and perform a number-one song on the Hot Country Songs chart. *Fearless* became the best-selling album of 2009 in the US. The album won four Grammy Awards, making Taylor he youngest Album of the Year winner.

As a singer-songwriter, Taylor has received awards from the Nashville Songwriters Association and the Songwriters

Hall of Fame. She was included in *Rolling Stone*'s 100 Greatest Songwriters of All Time in 2015. She has also received ten Grammys, one Emmy, 23 *Billboard* Music Awards, and 12 Country Music Association Awards. She currently holds six Guinness World Records. Taylor is one of the best-selling music artists of all time. She has sold over 40 million albums.

But when she was younger, she said she wouldn't get invited to birthday and other parties. She was picked on because she liked country music and wasn't considered pretty enough. In a *Teen Vogue* article, Taylor said that "Junior high was actually sort of hard because I got dumped by this group of popular girls...They didn't think I was cool or pretty enough, so they stopped talking to me. The kids at school thought it was weird that I liked country [music]," she says. "They'd make fun of me."[17]

At one point no one would sit with her at lunch, and the other kids branded her "weird."

In a *Heat World* article, her mom Andrea said, "My worst time of day was when I used to pick Taylor up from school. I would know things hadn't been great. Literally, the shunning that would take place at school – she would sit down at lunchtime and everyone would move."[18]

I love that Taylor's experiences didn't make her hard or lose sight of her dreams. And it seems the number one, award-winning song she co-wrote, *Shake It Off*, is really Taylor's philosophy to bullying. When a fan named Hannah tagged the singer in a photo on Instagram in 2014 and wrote how she was being picked on, here's what Taylor responded with:

"I hate thinking about your pretty face covered in tears, but I know why you're crying because I've been in your place. This isn't a high school thing or an age thing. It's a people thing. A life thing. It doesn't stop. It doesn't end or change. People cut other people down for entertainment, amusement, out of jealousy, because of something broken inside them. Or for no reason at all.

It's just what they do, and you're a target because you live your life loudly and boldly. You're bright and joyful and so many people are cynical. They won't understand you and they won't understand me. But the only way they win is if your tears turn to stone and make you bitter like them. It's okay to ask why. It's okay to wonder how you could try so hard and still get stomped all over. Just don't let them change you or stop you from singing or dancing around to your favorite song.

You're going into high school this week and this is your chance to push the reset button on how much value you give the opinion of these kids, most of whom have NO idea who they are. I'm so proud of you and protective of you because you DO. If they don't like you for being yourself, be yourself even more.

Every time someone picks on me, I'll think of you in the hopes that every time someone picks on you, you'll think of me... and how we have this thread that connects us. Let them keep living in the darkness and we'll keep walking in the sunlight. Forever on your side, Taylor."

What I learned from Taylor:

Don't give the bullies what they want by sobbing your heart out. Instead of letting "your tears turn to stone," shine as bright as you can.

What did you learn?

_____

_____

_____

_____

_____

#9

elon musk

Entrepreneur, Inventor

Elon Reeve Musk was born on June 28, 1971, in Pretoria, South Africa. Although he grew up in South Africa, Elon has been granted Canadian and US citizenship. Elon taught himself computer programming at the age of 10. He moved to Canada when he was 17 to attend university, and then transferred to the University of Pennsylvania.

Elon has made a career out of starting businesses that change the way we do things. He started an internet company that merged with PayPal, which changed the way we pay for things online. He took over an electric car company when electric cars were considered a silly dream and has built Tesla into a company that has changed the auto industry forever. He created another company, SpaceX, that launches rockets into space. He's actively working to reduce global warming through sustainable energy production and consumption and to establish a human colony on Mars.

But this iconic entrepreneur grew up being teased and physically abused. His mother, Maye Musk, said in an interview with *Esquire* magazine that Elon was "the youngest and smallest guy in his school" and that he was picked on all the time.[19] The abuse included him being thrown down a flight of stairs and beaten up so badly that he blacked out.

Elon survived the bullying in two ways. The first was by staying close with his family and embracing the risk-taking and adventurous tradition that apparently goes back generations. The other way was to become obsessed with business and technology, which led to his groundbreaking careers. By the time he was 17 he had already tried to start a business, a video arcade, but wasn't able to get the final permits required to open. But his ambition and work ethic led to his enormous successes. In 2016 *Forbes* magazine ranked him one of "The World's Most Powerful People."

What I learned from Elon:

Size doesn't matter, but the size of your brain and your dreams do. Elon was driven to do the things other kids told him he couldn't.

What did you learn?

_____

_____

_____

_____

_____

> **"The bully is the unhappiest person in the world at that moment."**
>
> - ZOE SALDANA

#10

zoe saldana

Actress, Philanthropist

Zoe Saldana-Perego was born Zoe Yadira Saldaña Nazario on June 19, 1978 in Passaic, New Jersey. Her father was from the Dominican Republic and her mother from Puerto Rico. She grew up mostly in Jackson Heights, New York and is bilingual in Spanish and English. Growing up she studied dance and performed with youth theatre groups in New York.

Her film breakthrough came when she got the role of Nyota Uhuru in 2009 in the *Star Trek* film series and the *Avatar* film series. Her long list of movie credits includes some of my favorite films, *Guardians of the Galaxy*, *Guardians of the Galaxy Vol. 2* and *Avengers: Infinity War* in 2018.

This gorgeous and talented actress was bullied as a child. In an *E! News* article Zoe discussed her childhood and how she dealt with the bullying that happened. "There was for a long time in my life when I was younger, I sort of gave up on trying to find female friends because girls can sometimes be a little too mean with each other. I don't know where it comes from, as opposed to us uniting, we tend to pick each other apart."[20]

But her mom helped her get through it.

"She never uplifted us by putting someone else down," Zoe recalled. "See, she would try to make us understand, look there is probably something going on in their lives, or you need to understand, as a person, nobody bullies when they're happy....So the bully is the unhappiest person around you at that moment. They're so unhappy he has to come and bother somebody else. Once you know all these things, and you know he is the one that feels most scared, the bully is the one that has very little regard for himself, very poor self-esteem."

I love what Zoe learned from this painful part of her life. "Once you understand that reality about a bully, you have won already. And you stick to the people that make you feel really good about yourself. But the one person that has to feel good about yourself is you. It takes practice...I look in the mirror... What are you going to do? You put something on. You practice the 'I'm beautiful. This is me. This is as good as it is going to get and it is great.'"

What I learned from Zoe:

I learned that once you understand the reality of a bully you have already won.

What did you learn?

_____

_____

_____

_____

_____

"Don't you ever let a soul in the world tell you that you can't be exactly who you are."

- LADY GAGA

#11

stefani germanotta

(Lady Gaga)

Singer, Songwriter, Actress, Philanthropist

Stefani Joanne Angelina Germanotta (Lady Gaga) was born March 28, 1986 in Manhattan, New York City. She learned to play the piano at age four. As a teenager Lady Gaga started playing music at open mic nights and acting in local theatre productions. She dropped out of the prestigious NYU Tisch School of the Arts to pursue music full time.

Today Lady Gaga is one of the best-selling music artists of all time. She's sold more than 27 million records and 146 million singles. She's received six Grammys and awards from both the Songwriters Hall of Fame and the Council of Fashion Designers of America. *Glamour* magazine named her Woman of the Year in 2013. She's adding to her list of acting credits, too. Lady Gaga won a Golden Globe Award in 2016 for Best Actress in a TV Miniseries or Film for her work on *American Horror Story*. Her performance in *A Star Is Born* earned her an Oscar nomination, and she won an Academy Award for co-writing a song in the film.

Lady Gaga was brutally bullied when she was younger and said she didn't fit in. She was teased for the size of her nose and for having buck teeth. She returned from gym class one day and discovered cuss words written all over her locker.

Talking about that period in her life, Lady Gaga told *Rolling Stone* in a 2011 article that the kids would say to her, "Your laugh is funny, you're weird, why do you always sing, why are you so into theater, why do you do your makeup like that, what's with your eyebrows?" They called her a "dyke" for the way she wore her hair and, she said, "I used to be called a slut."[21] It was so bad she didn't even want to go to school sometimes.

At her concert at Madison Square Garden in February of 2011, which was filmed and became an HBO special, Gaga told the audience that in high school she was thrown in the trash.[22] She was going to a pizzeria one day after school and some boys who were friends with girls who didn't like her attacked her.

"So the guys were like, let me put you in the trash where you belong. So they picked me up in my school skirt and they put me in the trash. And I remember I was looking up at them, and I was trying to laugh to act like it didn't bother me because I didn't want to show a sign of weakness. But really I was holding back the tears so hard because I was so embarrassed that I was in the trash can." She continued by encouraging her fans and anyone who has experienced being bullied, "I am living proof that if anyone ever puts you in a f***ing trash can, you can always get the f*** out."

Gaga had her teeth fixed. She worked on her music and passion. And she triumphed over those who tried to crush her. "When I did not believe in myself, when I was bullied in school, I felt ugly, and my only escape was music and that's why I started to sing and write songs and act. It was because I wanted an escape from all of that pain," Lady Gaga said in *Variety*.

Her experiences, and triumphing over them, helped inspire her to create a nonprofit, the Born This Way Foundation. The foundation works to empower and combat bullying through programs that enhance the mental wellness of youth and by working with organizations to empower young people to create a kinder, braver world. Because, as she said backstage at her filmed concert, "I feel like I'm fighting for every kid that's like me. That felt like I felt and feels like I still feel...It's not about me being a winner for me anymore. It's about being a winner for all of them."

What I learned from Lady Gaga:

You can always pick yourself up. Even if you were thrown in an effing trash can.

What did you learn?

_____

_____

_____

_____

_____

#12

mila kunis

Actress

Milena Markovna "Mila" Kunis was born on August 14, 1983 in Chernivtsi, Ukrainian SSR in the Soviet Union. In 1991, at the age of seven and in second grade, she moved from Soviet Ukraine to the United States with her family. When they arrived in Los Angeles with only $250 and a dream for a better life.

"I blocked out second grade completely," Mila said according to a Wikipedia article. "I have no recollection of it. I always talk to my Mom and my grandma about it. It was because I cried every day. I didn't understand the culture. I didn't understand the people. I didn't understand the language."[24]

Later, she enrolled in acting classes as an after-school activity, and she was soon discovered by a talent agent. She appeared in several television series and commercials before nabbing the role that would put her on the map at 14, playing Jackie Burkhart on the long-running TV series *That '70s Show*.

Since 1999, she's been the voice of Meg Griffin on the animated series *Family Guy* (one of my favorite shows). She's been in blockbuster movies including: *Forgetting Sarah Marshall*, *Friends with Benefits* and *Ted*. She's been nominated for Screen Actors Guild awards, Teen Choice Awards, People's Choice Awards, MTV Awards, and many more.

Even though Mila was named the "Sexiest Woman Alive" by *Esquire* magazine in 2013, she was bullied because of how she looked as a kid. She was always the smallest in her class and was constantly being made fun of for her big eyes, big lips and big ears. "I used to come home crying, 'Why do I have big eyes?' And my parents were like, 'You're crazy!" she said in a *Daily Mail* article. "I've learned it wasn't a bad thing to be picked on because when you're little it seems awful, like it's the end of the world. I grew into my face."[25]

What I learned from Mila:

The parts of your appearance that you get teased about can end up being some of the things people admire most.

What did you learn?

_____

_____

_____

_____

#13

robyn rihanna fenty

(Rhianna)

Singer, Actress, Diplomat, Businesswoman

Robyn Rihanna Fenty, known to the world as Rihanna, was born on February 20, 1988 in Saint Michael, Barbados, an island in the Caribbean Sea. Rihanna has been recognized as a pop, beauty and fashion icon. Her music accomplishments include nine Grammy Awards, 12 Billboard Music Awards, 12 American Music Awards and eight People's Choice Awards.

Her music has sold more than 10 million albums in the US alone, and she earned a Guinness World Record for achieving digital sales of more than 58 million in 2012. In the UK, she's sold more than 18 million singles and six million albums. Only the Beatles have sold more million-selling singles in the UK.

Her multimillion-dollar successes as an entrepreneur in the music industry, fashion and beauty are equally impressive. In 2013 Rihanna collaborated with MAC Cosmetics and released her own line of makeup called "RiRi hearts MAC."

In 2014 Puma named her the creative director for their women's collections, driving Puma's sales through the roof. She's a co-owner of the music streaming company, Tidal, and her own beauty and stylist agency. Her insanely successful Fenty Beauty and Savage clothing and accessories brands focus on diversity and inclusiveness, which the sales show her fans want.

I was surprised that someone who now dominates several industries was brutally teased as a kid. In a *Glamour* magazine interview, she shared how other students at her school used to bully her. She was teased about many things, from the size of her breasts to the color of her skin because it was lighter than her classmates.

"I got teased my entire school life. What they were picking on I don't even understand," Rihanna said. "It was my skin color. Then when I got older, it was about my breasts. But I'm not victimized—I'm grateful. I think those experiences were strategically put together by God for the preparation of being in the music industry. It's so easy for me to deal with the [challenges] now."[26]

What I learned from Rihanna:

You may look different. So what if you do? You are beautiful no matter what.

What did you learn?

_____

_____

_____

_____

_____

"**People are going to bring you down because of your drive. Ultimately, it makes you a stronger person to turn your cheek and go the other way.**"

- SELENA GOMEZ

#14

jennifer lawrence

Actress, Activist, Philanthropist

Jennifer Shrader Lawrence was born on August 15, 1990 in Indian Hills, Kentucky. As a girl she felt like a misfit and like she didn't fit in.

While on vacation in New York, a talent scout saw her walking down the street. He arranged for her to audition to talent agents, which led to her epic acting career.

She began her career acting with appearances on television shows, and at 18 started getting roles in movies. She's appeared in more than 35 movies and television shows, including two "mega-franchises," *The Hunger Games* and *X-Men*. In 2012 she was awarded the Academy Award for Best Actress for her performance in *Silver Linings Playbook*, the second youngest winner in the history of the category. Her films have earned nearly six billion dollars worldwide, making her one of the highest-paid actresses in the world. According to *Forbes*, she topped the list in 2015 and 2016.

Jennifer is passionate about many causes outside of acting that focus on access to healthcare, women's equality and kids. In 2015 she started the Jennifer Lawrence Foundation that supports charities like the Boys & Girls Clubs of America and the Special Olympics. She donated millions of dollars to start a cardiac intensive care unit at the Kosair Children's Hospital in Louisville.

She's also involved with Represent.Us, a nonprofit working to pass anti-corruption laws in the United States. And she's been involved with Time's Up, a movement to fight against harassment and discrimination against women.

After learning about her experience being bullied, it's easy to understand why she's so active in causes that focus on making sure people aren't left out or discriminated against. Growing up, Jennifer was a tomboy and even played on the boys' basketball team, which made her an easy target for bullying.

She was picked on and excluded by other girls. "I changed schools a lot when I was in elementary school because some girls were mean," Jennifer revealed in an interview with *The Sun*. She said, "Don't worry about the bitches. That could be a good motto, because you come across people like that throughout your life."[27]

What I learned from Jennifer:

If you are different, don't be afraid to shine! Stand out and be a trailblazer.

What did you learn?

_____

_____

_____

_____

_____

> **"People who love themselves, don't hurt other people. The more we hate ourselves, the more we want others to suffer."**
>
> - DAN PEARCE

#15

tom cruise

Actor, Producer

Thomas Cruise Mapother IV was born on July 3, 1962 in Syracuse, New York. He began acting when he was 19 years old. Tom has been in more than 50 movies, including *Risky Business, Rain Man, A Few Good Men* and the *Mission Impossible* movies. His films have earned $10 billion globally, and he's considered one of the most powerful men in Hollywood.

Tom grew up far away from the wealthy, Hollywood-star life he now lives. He lived in near-poverty, was small for his age, and struggled with reading, which forced him into special classes and made him a social outcast. He moved to 15 different schools over 12 years and suffered from bullying.

The abuse wasn't just at school, but also inside his home. Tom once called his father, who beat him growing up, "a merchant of chaos" and "a bully and coward."[28]

"He was the kind of person where, if something goes wrong, they kick you," Tom said. "It was a great lesson in my life—how he'd lull you in, make you feel safe and then, bang! For me, it was like, 'There's something wrong with this guy. Don't trust him. Be careful around him.'"

Tom said, "So many times the big bully comes up, pushes me," he recalled. "Your heart's pounding, you sweat, and you feel like you're going to vomit...I don't like bullies."

Tom reunited with his father when he was in the hospital dying of cancer. His dad would only meet him if Tom agreed not to ask him anything about the past. "When I saw him in pain, I thought, 'Wow, what a lonely life,'" Tom said. "He was in his late 40s. It was sad."

What I learned from Tom:

First, if he could forgive his dad, I can certainly forgive my bullies. And second, I identify a lot with Tom because he was small for his age and was teased for it. Yet he still became a larger-than-life figure.

What did you learn?

_____

_____

_____

_____

_____

#16

pierce brosnan

Actor, Film Producer, Activist

Pierce Brendan Brosnan OBE was born May 16, 1953 in Drogheda, Ireland, and he had a challenging childhood When he was an infant, his father abandoned his family. At four, his mother moved to London and he was raised by his grandparents. After their death he was sent to a boarding school.

He left school when he was 16 years old and started working as a painter. Pierce started attending the Saint Martin's School of Art to learn how to be an illustrator for companies. I learned that people in this career make drawings, images, paintings or diagrams for products. But his time there didn't last long.

He left and worked in the circus for a few years, before returning to study drama. Pierce fell in love with acting and made it his career. He began acting in plays and, a few years later, started to get small roles in films.

In the early 1980s he moved from England to Southern California and worked first in television. For five years he was on the hit television series, *Remington Steele* before moving into movies. He's been in nine television shows and more than 65 movies. His movie credits include playing James Bond four times in *GoldenEye, Tomorrow Never Dies, The World is Not Enough* and *Die Another Day*. He's also had starring roles in *Mrs. Doubtfire* (where I got introduced to him), *Mamma Mia!* and the sequel, *Mamma Mia! Here We Go Again.*

If you're wondering what the OBE in Pierce's name means, it stands for Order of the British Empire. It's an award he received for his work in drama and movies. The Queen of England gave it to him.

Growing up Pierce was discriminated against and teased at school because he was different from other kids. In a *Chicago Tribune* article he said, "Trying to fit in then in 1964 in the English comprehensive school system was not easy. So being the token Irish lad [in school in England] was not easy. There was a certain discrimination, and I was the butt of quite a few jokes. They could never find the way to say my name or couldn't say my name, or didn't want to say the name, 'Pierce', so I was known as 'Irish' throughout my years. And I wore that as a badge and an emblem of great dignity. I liked the mystique of it. You learn at an early age to roll with the punches and find your way through the day [with] a sense of humor," he said.[29] According to Pierce's IMDb biography, he was six feet tall by the time he was 11, which also led to teasing.

What I learned from Pierce:

Take what you're being bullied about and turn it into a badge of honor. And if this leading man was teased for being too tall that I shouldn't feel badly about being teased for being short. If someone wants to bully you, they'll find a reason!

What did you learn?

_____

_____

_____

_____

_____

"When people hurt you over and over, think of them like sand paper. They may scratch and hurt you a bit, but in the end, you end up polished and they end up useless."

- CHRIS COLFER

#17

chris colfer

Actor, Singer, Author, Philanthropist

Christopher Paul Colfer was born May 27, 1990 in Clovis, California. Colfer, who had always wanted to be an actor and had joined a local dinner theater ensemble at age 11, became active in theater and debate.

He had a main role in the television series *Glee* playing gay teen Kurt Hummel from 2009-2015. He's also appeared on *Saturday Night Live*, *Entertainment Tonight* and *RuPaul's Drag Race: All Stars*. Chris has appeared in seven movies, including *Marmaduke*, *Glee: the 3D Concert Movie* and *Absolutely Fabulous: The Movie*.

Over the years he's won more than 20 awards for his work. They include seven Teen Choice Awards, five Screen Actors Guild Awards, four People's Choice Awards and two Primetime Emmy Awards.

In addition to acting, this multi-talented, openly gay star also wrote, directed and acted in the movie *Struck by Lightning* and wrote an episode of *Glee*. Chris has also written several books, including *Stranger than Fanfiction* and *The New York Times* number-one best-selling book *The Land of Stories: The Wishing Spell*, which is the first in a series of 11 novels for middle schoolers.

Chris supports nonprofits that help people improve their lives. He's an active supporter of the It Gets Better Campaign and The Trevor Project, two nonprofits that work to prevent suicide among lesbian, gay, bisexual, transgender, and questioning (LGBTQ) kids. For two years in a row, he was also the co-chair for the Elton John AIDS Foundation Academy Award Party.

He's been involved in raising awareness of the importance of animal adoption and children's literacy. In 2015 he donated all of the profits from the sales of T-shirts with quotes from his *The Land of Stories* books series to benefit First Book, a nonprofit that gives new books to kids in need.

Chris had to overcome a lot to get where he is today. He was home-schooled for most of middle school because he was getting bullied so badly. In a 2011 interview for *Entertainment*, he said, "I was very tiny. I spent most of my time stuffed into lockers. Thank god for cell phones, or I'd still be in there."[30]

He returned to public school for high school. "I went to a school much worse than McKinley," where Kurt and the other *Glee* kids attend, Chris said. "I wasn't honest with myself in high school" because the constant bullying convinced him he "couldn't get lower" than being gay.

Chris credits his forensics coach, Mikendra McCoy, with helping him love who he was. She told him, "If you own who you are, no one can hold *you* against you." He took that advice to heart and developed his sense of humor that became Kurt's and that fans love.

The role of Kurt was written specifically for Chris. For example, boys would yell at Kurt in the show, "Hey, what's sex with men like?" And he'd shoot back, "Don't you remember?"

What I learned from Chris:

Turn something bad into inspiration. Also, don't forget to whip in some quick and witty humor.

What did you learn?

_____

_____

_____

_____

_____

"Never be bullied into silence. Never allow yourself to be made a victim. Accept no one's definition of your life; define yourself."

- HARVEY FIERSTEIN

#18

jesse tyler ferguson

Actor, Singer, Philanthropist

Jesse Tyler Ferguson was born October 22, 1975 in Missoula, Montana, but raised mostly in Albuquerque, New Mexico. He had an interest in acting from a young age. At eight years old he joined the Albuquerque Children's Theatre. He also had roles in his high school's plays and was in the speech and debate team. He went to the prestigious The American Musical and Dramatic Academy (AMDA) in New York City for college.

Jesse has appeared in nine movies, 18 television shows and 17 theatre productions. His most famous role, and where I first saw him, is on the television show *Modern Family*, which has been on the air for nine years. He's received six Screen Actors Guild Awards, five Primetime Emmy Awards and two People's Choice Awards.

Growing up he was bullied because kids suspected he was gay. He was kicked, got his hair pulled and ate alone in the lunchroom. He had horrible grades because he couldn't focus. "I feel like I was cheated of an education too because I was so worried about keeping myself safe," Jesse said in an interview with *TV Guide*.[31] Even though he had to change high schools because of bullying, he kept his focus on the big picture.

"One thing that got me through that time was knowing that there's a much larger world outside of high school," Jesse said. "Four years is a really long when you're a kid and being bullied, but to know that I had 50 or 60 years outside of high school where I was going to live the life I was going to live and not worry about bullies was huge for me."

Jesse told Oprah Winfrey in an episode of her *Master Class* show, "Being bullied shaped my character. It made me a stronger person. It made me want to succeed. Everything they tried to knock me down for made me want to climb out and want to achieve those things."[32]

What I learned from Jesse:

Be who you are. Be proud of who you are and don't try and hide it.

What did you learn?

_____

_____

_____

_____

_____

"Don't let it get to you. Just know at the end of the day, you are strong and there are people that love you even if sometimes it doesn't feel like it. It always gets better."

- BETHANY MOTA

#19

patrick ta

Makeup Artist to the Stars

Patrick Ta was born February 12, 1991, in San Diego California. He began doing makeup when he was young. In a People magazine interview, he shared how he taught himself how to do make up by watching YouTube videos.[33]

Now Patrick is a makeup artist for high-profile celebrities. His friends and clients include Ariana Grande, Olivia Munn, Sofia Carson, and Chrissy Teigen. After only six years in his career, one of the biggest makeup companies in the world chose him to be its Global Makeup Colour Artist. With more than a million Instagram followers, he's one of the go-to artists in the industry.

But before he was a famous makeup artist and surrounded by celebrities, he was a kid who was horrendously bullied. In fact, the bullying was so bad he dropped out of high school.

"I was called so many names. So many. Fatty, Fatty Patty, Fatrick and I didn't deal with it very well," Patrick told *Glamour* magazine.[34]

The bullying caused him to feel "super unconfident" for most of life. "I'll always feel like Fatty Patty on some level." His lack of confidence finally started to change when he got successful in his career, and it was about his skill and not his appearance. Patrick totally sees the irony in how he's found success in making other people look beautiful, while his childhood was so hard because people said he looked so ugly. "It goes to show that makeup and beauty go so much deeper in so many ways."

Patrick has been open about his bullying on social media, and he's received messages from parents with pictures of their kids going through similar experiences that have made him cry. One mom even had her son read Patrick's post out loud so he'd believe this phase in his life would pass and the future would be brighter.

He has a powerful message for anyone being bullied. "I think it really helps to discover what you're passionate about and what inspires you and focus on that rather than the bullies. If you pursue your passion, you'll shine and prove all those bullies wrong in the end."

What I learned from Patrick:

Focus on what you love and being you. Because that's how I will find success and be celebrated for what I am instead of being bullied for what I'm not.

What did you learn?

_____

_____

_____

_____

_____

"You are not alone in this. There are so many people going through the same thing. Just know that you are stronger than any voice that brings you down."

- BRITTANY SNOW

#20

I've found this whole process of writing my story and thinking about the lessons I've learned to be really helpful and therapeutic. So I wanted to give you the chance to do it too. I totally get that you're not famous....yet. Even so, you're #20.

I want you to write your story and the lessons you've learned, and then be brave enough to share it with others. I know you can help them, and sharing it will help you, like it has me.

What is your story?

_____

_____

_____

_____

_____

_____

_____

_____

_____

_____

_____

_____

_____

_____

_____

_____

_____

_____

_____

_____

_____

_____

_____

What did you (or are you) learning?

_____

_____

_____

_____

_____

_____

_____

acknowledgments

I would like to thank my English teachers, Mrs. Heyde, Mrs. Rosenberg, and Mrs. Goldblatt for helping me improve my writing and express my feelings on the page. I'd like to thank my Journalism class and Mrs. Goldblatt for teaching me how to fact find and report on issues I'm interested in. Thank you to my sister for supporting me during this process. Thank you to my grandparents—Bubbie, Grandpa and Grandma—for always supporting and loving me.

I am especially thankful for my parents who have not only supported me but encouraged me to step (leap, really) outside my comfort zone to do a Bar Mitzvah project that really stretched and scared me. They were not only my editors and strategic team, they supported me every step of the way. Like they always do.

Last but not least, I would like to thank the bullies. Without them, I would have never written this book. You've made me stronger, and I'm grateful.

bullying by the numbers

These statistics are provided by Stopbullying.gov and stompoutbullying.org.

Bullying stats:

- One out of four kids is bullied.

- Every seven seconds a child is bullied.

- Depending on the age group, up to 43% of students say they have been digitally harassed.

- 5.4 million students skip school at some point in the year due to bullying.

- Nine out of ten LGBT students experienced harassment at school.

- Child and teen Bullying and Cyberbullying are both a growing problem.

- Some kids are so tormented that suicide has become an alternative for them. However, most suicides are not just a result of bullying. There are usually other factors involved.

- Being a bully can mess up their own future. Bullies are more likely to skip school, drop out of school, smoke, drink alcohol, get into fights and be arrested at some point in their life. Sixty percent of boys who were bullies in middle school had at least one criminal conviction by the age of 24.

- Seventy-seven percent of students are bullied mentally, verbally, and physically. Cyberbullying statistics are rapidly approaching similar numbers, with 43% experiencing cyberbullying.

- Of the 77% of students that said they had been bullied, 14% of those who were bullied said they experienced severe (bad) reactions to the abuse.

- One in five students admit to being a bully, or doing some "Bullying."

- Each day 160,000 students miss school for fear of being bullied.

- Forty-three percent of kids fear harassment in the bathroom at school.

- One hundred thousand students carry a gun to school.

- Twenty-eight percent of youths who carry weapons have witnessed violence at home.

- Two hundred eighty-two thousand students are physically attacked in secondary schools each month.

- More youth violence occurs on school grounds than happens on the way to school.

- Playground school bullying statistics:

    ○ Every seven seconds a child is bullied.

    ○ Adults intervene four percent of the time.

    ○ Peers intervene 11% of the time.

    ○ Eighty-five percent of the time no one intervenes.

- Thirty percent of U.S. students in grades six through ten are involved in moderate or frequent bullying—as bullies, as victims, or as both—according to the results of the first national school bullying statistics and cyberbullying statistics survey on this subject.

- School bullying and cyberbullying are increasingly viewed as important contributors to youth violence, including homicide and suicide.

- Case studies of the shooting at Columbine High School and other U.S. schools suggest that bullying was a factor in many of the incidents.

helpful resources

National Suicide Prevention Hotline

The National Suicide Prevention Hotline's mission is to "Help prevent suicide. The Lifeline provides 24/7, free and confidential support for people in distress, prevention and crisis resources for you or your loved ones, and best practices for professionals."

The Suicide Prevention Hotline number is: **1-800-273-8255**
https://suicidepreventionlifeline.org

Born This Way Foundation

Founded by Lady Gaga, the foundation works to empower and combat bullying through programs that enhance the mental wellness of youth and by working with organizations to empower young people to create a kinder, braver world.

https://bornthisway.foundation

Kind Campaign

The Kind Campaign was started in 2009 by Lauren Parsekian and Molly Thompson. They were both bullied by girls. They created a documentary and non-profit to stop what they call "girl on girl crime."

https://www.kindcampaign.com

The Trevor Project

This organization provides support to LGBTQ youth over the phone, online, and through a texting. They have a 24/7 crisis intervention and suicide prevention phone service you can call for help anytime at 866-488-7386. Their confidential, instant messaging chat service can be accessed through a computer from their website, https://www.thetrevorproject. org. And they have confidential text messaging. Simply text START to 678678.

https://www.thetrevorproject.org

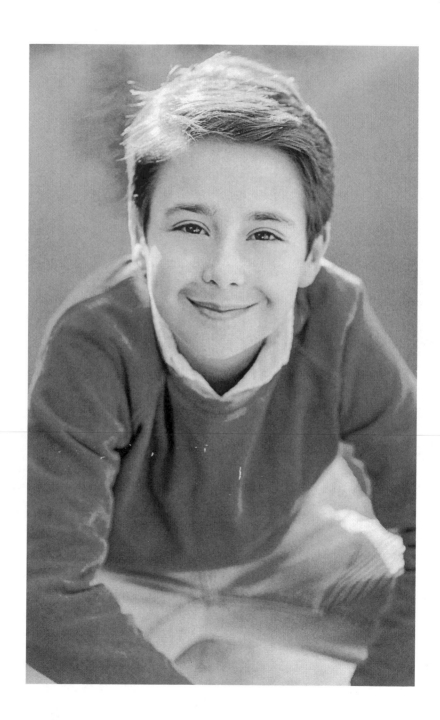

about the author

In case you want to know a little more about me, here it is. I'm 14 years old and in 8th grade. I was born in Bozeman, Montana and moved to sunny San Diego when I was six. My favorite subjects in school are journalism, history, and music, and I'm also on the school tennis team. I love acting, singing, tennis, reading, cooking, video games and following club soccer. One of my biggest passions is traveling to other countries to explore the culture and the food. I study dance, acting and voice, and have appeared in local youth theatre productions of *Les Miserable*, *The Lion King* and *Seussical*, among others. I live at home with my mom Romi, my dad John, my sister Bebe and Sadie, our Australian labradoodle.

references

1. Facts About Bullying. U.S. Department of Health and Human Services. https://www.stopbullying.gov/media/facts/index.html#ftn2. Accessed October 19, 2018.

2. E. DeGeneres, Web Exclusive: Justin Timberlake on Bullying, *The Ellen Show*, November 10, 2010, https://youtu.be/JLhvTcEWbEg, (accessed July 28, 2019).

3. Justin Timberlake's Acceptance Speech | iHeart Radio Music Awards 2017, *iHeartRadio*, March 5, 2017, https://youtu.be/buXwsEjlgXU, (accessed July 28, 2019).

4. R. Adams, Tyra Banks Talks Weight & Self-Esteem On HuffPost Live (VIDEO), *HuffPost News*, September 17, 2012, https://www.huffpost.com/entry/tyra-banks-weight-self-esteem-girls-club-interview_n_1886465, (accessed July 28, 2019).

5. T. Banks, "Confessions of a Former Mean Girl," *Teen People*, August 2005, pg. 52.

6. #568 Steven Spielberg, *Forbes*, July 28, 2019, https://www.forbes.com/profile/steven-spielberg/#3180e073228a, (accessed July 28, 2019).

7. T. Shone, Steven Spielberg: 'It's all about making kids feel like they can do anything', *The Guardian*, July 16, 2016, https://www.theguardian.com/film/2016/jul/16/steven-spielberg-kids-can-do-anything-bfg, (accessed July 28, 2019).

8. B. Weinraud, FILM; Steven Spielberg Faces the Holocaust, *The New York Times*, December 12, 1993, https://www.nytimes.com/1993/12/12/movies/film-steven-spielberg-faces-the-holocaust.html, (accessed July 28, 2019).

9. S. Dubner, Steven the Good, *New York Times Magazine*, February 14, 1999, https://www.nytimes.com/1999/02/14/magazine/steven-the-good.html, (accessed July 28, 2019).

10. P. Gicas. Steven Spielberg Reveals He Was Bullied as a Child, *E! News*, October 22, 2012, https://www.eonline.com/news/355970/steven-spielberg-reveals-he-was-bullied-as-a-child, (accessed July 28, 2019).

11. D. Feldmann, Spielberg, Steven, *Learning to Give*, https://www.learningtogive.org/resources/spielberg-steven, (accessed July 28, 2019).

12. S. Hollis, The rise, fall, and rise again of The Honest Company, *Upsell*, July 19, 2018, https://jilt.com/blog/honest-company-adversity, (accessed July 28, 2019).

13. T.L. Croom, *Diary of a Bullied Child: Smell of Stardom*. Bloomington, IN: WestBow Press; 2011.

14. Michael Phelps shares being bullied, depressed in film, *NBC Sports*, October 11,

2017, https://olympics.nbcsports.com/2017/10/11/michael-phelps-angst-film-clip-video/, (accessed July 28, 2019).

15. P. Forde, Michael Phelps turns tables on childhood bullies, *Yahoo! Sports*, July 27, 2012, https://www.yahoo.com/news/olympics--michael-phelps-turns-tables-on-childhood-bullies.html, (accessed July 28, 2019).

16. S. People, I took beatings from several boys at school for years.. but it made me tough enough to stand up to DiCaprio and get my big break.., *Mirror*, February 10, 2013, https://www.mirror.co.uk/news/world-news/i-took-beatings-from-several-boys-at-school-1655646, (accessed July 28, 2019).

17. L. Waterman, Swift Ascent, *Teen Vogue*, January 25, 2009, https://www.teenvogue.com/story/teen-vogue-cover-girl-taylor-swift_090126/amp, (accessed July 28, 2019).

18. E. Saunders, EXCLUSIVE: How Taylor Swift overcame BULLYING and fat-shaming to become the world's biggest pop star, *Heat World*, February 24, 2015, https://heatworld.com/celebrity/news/exclusive-taylor-swift-overcame-bullying-fat-shaming-become-world-s-biggest-pop/, (accessed July 28, 2019).

19. T. Junod, Elon Musk: Triumph of His Will, *Esquire*, November 15, 2012, https://www.esquire.com/news-politics/a16681/elon-musk-interview-1212/, (accessed July 29, 2019).

20. B. Nessif, Pregnant Zoe Saldana Recalls Hating "Girly" Things as a Kid, Talks About Being Bullied—Watch Now, *E! Online*, October 21, 2014, https://www.eonline.com/news/590604/pregnant-zoe-saldana-recalls-hating-girly-things-as-a-kid-talks-about-being-bullied-watch-now, (accessed July 28, 2019).

21. B. Hiatt, Deep Inside the Unreal World of Lady Gaga, *Rolling Stone*, June 9, 2011, https://www.rollingstone.com/music/music-news/deep-inside-the-unreal-world-of-lady-gaga-86008/, (accessed July 28, 2019).

22. Lady Gaga Presents the Monster Ball Tour: At Madison Square Garden, May 17, 2011, https://youtu.be/e6ZdtGI75IQ, (accessed July 28, 2019).

23. Lady Gaga Recalls Being Bullied in School: 'I Felt Ugly'. *Variety*. https://variety.com/video/lady-gaga-bradley-cooper-star-is-born-bullied/. Accessed July 28, 2019.

24. Mila Kunis. *Wikipedia*. https://en.wikipedia.org/wiki/Mila_Kunis. Accessed July 28, 2019.

25. 'I was bullied at school over my funny-looking face,' reveals Black Swan beauty Mila Kunis. *Daily Mail*. 2011. https://www.dailymail.co.uk/tvshowbiz/article-1355984/I-bullied-school-funny-looking-face-reveals-Black-Swan-beauty-Mila-Kunis.html. Accessed July 28, 2019.

26. The Difference Between Robyn and Rihanna, According to Rihanna, *Glamour*,

October 1, 2013, https://www.glamour.com/story/the-difference-between-robyn-a, accessed July 28, 2019.

27. Jennifer Lawrence Bullied: Oscar Winner Admits To Being The Unpopular Girl In Middle School, *HuffPost*, March 7, 2013, https://www.huffingtonpost.com/2013/03/07/jennifer-lawrence-bullied_n_2830763.html, (accessed July 28, 2019).

28. Tom Cruise says his father was 'a bully', *Today Celebrities*, April 5, 2006, http://www.today.com/id/12171938/ns/today-today_entertainment/t/tom-cruise-says-his-father-was-bully/#.W8UgwhNKjOQ, (accessed July 28, 2019).

29. Lee L. Amid tragedy, Brosnan leans on faith and work. http://digitaledition.chicagotribune.com/tribune/article_popover.aspx?guid=cdba4cf6-944f-466a-9d6f-9879b64e854f. Accessed October 1, 2018.

30. L. Beard, Chris Colfer of "Glee" talks bullying, *Entertainment*, October 3, 2011, https://ew.com/article/2011/10/03/chris-colfer-glee-new-yorker-festival/, (accessed July 28, 2019).

31. N. Abrams, Modern Family's Jesse Tyler Ferguson: I Left School (Because of Bullying), *TV Guide*, October 9, 2010, https://www.tvguide.com/news/modern-familys-ferguson-1024173/, (accessed July 28, 2019).

32. How Being Bullied Made Jesse Tyler Ferguson Stronger, *OWN*, October 22, 2015, https://youtu.be/wL75QOPXHC8, (accessed July 28, 2019).

33. J. Ruffo, The Pro Files: How Patrick Ta Went from Working at M.A.C. to Top Celebrity Makeup Artist in 4 Years, *People*, February 15, 2018, https://people.com/style/how-makeup-artist-patrick-ta-got-his-start/, (accessed July 28, 2019).

34. L. Winter, Ariana Grande's makeup artist, Patrick Ta, reveals he dropped out of school after being so badly bullied, *Glamour*, October 7, 2018, https://www.glamourmagazine.co.uk/article/patrick-ta-anti-bullying, (accessed July 28, 2019).

Made in the USA
San Bernardino, CA
11 September 2019